MW00883573

PREVENT
AND
REVERSE
HEART DISEASE
COOKBOO
K

Delicious Recipes
For A Heart-
Healthy Lifestyle

BINAMIN

COPYRIGHT

MY STORY

My journey towards writing this book began with a deeply personal experience. Several years ago, a close family member was diagnosed with heart disease. The news came as a shock to all of us, and we were suddenly thrust into a world of medical jargon, doctor's appointments, and a pressing need to make significant lifestyle changes. As we navigated this new reality, I quickly realized that there was a vast amount of information available but little that was easily accessible or practical for someone just starting out.

My background is in nutrition, and I have always been passionate about the power of food to heal and nourish the body. However, even with my professional knowledge, I found it challenging to sift through the myriad of dietary recommendations and conflicting advice. What my family needed was clear, concise guidance and practical tools to make heart-healthy eating a part of our daily lives. This experience ignited a desire in me to create a resource that could help others in similar situations.

I began researching extensively, consulting with cardiologists, dietitians, and other experts in the field of heart health. I wanted to ensure that the information and recipes I provided were not only accurate but also easy to implement and enjoyable. Over time, I started compiling recipes that were both heart-healthy and delicious, experimenting with different ingredients and cooking techniques to create meals that were satisfying and nutritious.

One of the biggest challenges we faced was finding meals that the whole family could enjoy. It was essential to me that the recipes in this book would appeal to a wide range of tastes and dietary preferences, ensuring that heart-healthy eating could be a family affair rather than an isolated effort. This book is the culmination of years of research, personal experience, and a deep commitment to helping others navigate the complexities of heart disease with confidence and ease.

Writing this book has been a labor of love. It is my hope that it will serve as a valuable resource for anyone newly diagnosed with heart disease, providing the knowledge and tools needed to make positive changes to their diet and lifestyle. I believe that with the right information and support, anyone can take control of their heart health and live a full, vibrant life.

In the pages that follow, you will find a wealth of information and delicious recipes designed to support your heart health. Whether you are looking for simple, everyday meals or dishes for special occasions, this book has something for everyone. I invite you to join me on this journey towards better heart health, one meal at a time. Let's cook, eat, and live heart-healthy together.

Heart disease is a term that encompasses various conditions affecting the heart, including coronary artery disease, heart rhythm problems, and heart defects, among others. It is one of the leading causes of death worldwide, but many forms of heart disease can be prevented or managed through lifestyle changes, particularly diet. This book will help you understand the role of nutrition in heart health and how to make the necessary changes to your diet without feeling deprived or overwhelmed.

We will explore the key nutrients that support heart health, the foods to avoid, and how to create balanced, satisfying meals. Whether you are new to cooking or an experienced home chef, this book offers something for everyone, with recipes that are both easy to follow and delicious. From quick breakfasts to hearty dinners and even indulgent desserts, you will find a wide range of options that cater to your taste buds and health needs.

INTRODUCTION

Understanding Heart Disease

Before we dive into the recipes and meal plans, it's essential to understand what heart disease is and why it requires such a dedicated approach to nutrition. Heart disease refers to various conditions that affect the heart's structure and function. The most common type is coronary artery disease, which occurs when the arteries that supply blood to the heart muscle become narrowed or blocked. This can lead to chest pain, heart attacks, and other serious complications.

Other forms of heart disease include heart valve disease, arrhythmias (irregular heartbeats), heart failure, and congenital heart defects. While some forms of heart disease are genetic, many are influenced by lifestyle factors such as diet, physical activity, and smoking. Therefore, making informed choices about what you eat can significantly impact your heart health and overall well-being.

Diet plays a crucial role in managing heart disease. Consuming a diet high in saturated fats, trans fats, cholesterol, and sodium can contribute to the development of heart disease by raising blood cholesterol levels and blood pressure. On the other hand, a diet rich in fruits, vegetables, whole grains, lean proteins, and healthy fats can help lower the risk of heart disease and improve heart health. This book will guide you in making these heart-healthy choices and show you how to enjoy a varied and flavorful diet.

How to Use This Book

This book is structured to provide you with a step-by-step approach to adopting a heart-healthy diet. We start with the basics of heart-healthy eating, discussing the essential nutrients and foods that support heart health and those that should be limited or avoided. Next, we guide you through meal planning and grocery shopping, offering tips on how to create balanced meal plans and navigate the grocery store to find heart-healthy ingredients.

The core of the book is the recipe sections, which are divided into breakfasts, lunches, dinners, snacks, desserts, and drinks. Each recipe includes detailed instructions, nutritional information, and tips for making the dish even healthier. Whether you are looking for quick weekday meals or recipes for special occasions, you will find plenty of inspiration here.

In addition to the recipes, we provide practical advice on lifestyle changes that support heart health, including physical activity and stress management. The final chapters of the book focus on creating sustainable habits and finding resources and support to help you on your journey.

Use this book as a tool to empower yourself with the knowledge and skills to make heart-healthy choices. Whether you are newly diagnosed or supporting a loved one, this book is here to help you every step of the way.

Overview of Heart Disease and Its Types

Heart disease is a term that covers a broad spectrum of conditions affecting the heart and its ability to function properly. It is one of the leading causes of death globally, accounting for millions of deaths each year. The term encompasses a variety of disorders that can affect the heart's structure, function, and blood vessels. Understanding these conditions is crucial for managing heart disease effectively, particularly through dietary and lifestyle changes.

1. Coronary Artery Disease (CAD):

- **Definition:** CAD is the most common type of heart disease. It occurs when the coronary arteries, which supply blood to the heart muscle, become narrowed or blocked due to the buildup of plaque (atherosclerosis).

- **Symptoms:** Common symptoms include chest pain (angina), shortness of breath, and fatigue. In severe cases, it can lead to heart attacks.

- **Causes:** The primary cause is the accumulation of fatty deposits on the artery walls, influenced by factors such as poor diet, lack of exercise, smoking, and high cholesterol.

2. Heart Failure:

- **Definition:** Heart failure, also known as congestive heart failure, occurs when the heart is unable to pump blood effectively to meet the body's needs.

- **Symptoms:** Symptoms include shortness of breath, fatigue, swollen legs, and rapid heartbeat. It can be chronic or acute.

- **Causes:** Causes include CAD, high blood pressure, previous heart attacks, and cardiomyopathy (disease of the heart muscle).

3. Arrhythmias:

- **Definition:** Arrhythmias are irregular heartbeats, which can be too fast (tachycardia), too slow (bradycardia), or erratic.

- **Symptoms:** Symptoms may include palpitations, dizziness, fainting, and shortness of breath.

- **Causes:** Causes include heart disease, electrolyte imbalances, injury from a heart attack, and congenital heart conditions.

4. Heart Valve Disease:

- **Definition:** This condition involves damage to one or more of the heart's valves, affecting how blood flows through the heart.

- **Symptoms:** Symptoms include fatigue, shortness of breath, and swelling in the ankles and feet.

- **Causes:** Causes include rheumatic fever, infections, congenital valve defects, and aging.

5. Cardiomyopathy:

- **Definition:** Cardiomyopathy refers to diseases of the heart muscle that make it harder for the heart to pump blood.

- **Symptoms:** Symptoms can include fatigue, shortness of breath, and swelling. It can lead to heart failure.

- **Causes:** Causes include genetic factors, long-term high blood pressure, heart tissue damage from a heart attack, and chronic rapid heart rate.

6. Congenital Heart Disease:

- **Definition:** Congenital heart disease refers to heart abnormalities present at birth.

- **Symptoms:** Symptoms vary widely depending on the type and severity of the defect and can include breathing difficulties, cyanosis (bluish tint to the skin), and poor weight gain.

- **Causes:** These defects arise from the heart's improper development in the womb due to genetic and environmental factors.

7. Peripheral Artery Disease (PAD):

- **Definition:** PAD occurs when the arteries that supply blood to the limbs, usually the legs, become narrowed or blocked.

- **Symptoms:** Symptoms include leg pain when walking (claudication), numbness, and weak pulse in the legs or feet.

- **Causes:** Similar to CAD, the primary cause is atherosclerosis.

Each type of heart disease requires specific management strategies, but many share common risk factors, including high blood pressure, high cholesterol, smoking, diabetes, obesity, and physical inactivity. Addressing these risk factors through diet and lifestyle changes can significantly impact the prevention and management of heart disease.

Importance of Diet and Lifestyle in Managing Heart Disease

Managing heart disease effectively often involves a combination of medical treatment and lifestyle changes. Among these, diet plays a crucial role. A heart-healthy diet can help manage risk factors such as high blood pressure, high cholesterol, and obesity, all of which contribute to heart disease.

1. Diet and Heart Disease:

- **Balanced Nutrition:** A balanced diet provides essential nutrients that support overall health and heart function. Key components include fruits, vegetables, whole grains, lean proteins, and healthy fats.

- **Reducing Saturated and Trans Fats:** High intake of saturated and trans fats can raise blood cholesterol levels, increasing the risk of CAD. Replacing these fats with unsaturated fats from sources like olive oil, nuts, and avocados can help lower cholesterol levels.

- **Limiting Sodium:** High sodium intake is linked to high blood pressure, a major risk factor for heart disease. Reducing sodium intake by avoiding processed foods and choosing fresh ingredients can help manage blood pressure.

- **Increasing Fiber Intake:** Dietary fiber, particularly soluble fiber, helps reduce cholesterol levels. Foods rich in fiber include fruits, vegetables, whole grains, and legumes.

- **Choosing Heart-Healthy Proteins:** Lean meats, fish, plant-based proteins, and low-fat dairy products provide essential nutrients without excessive saturated fats. Fish, especially fatty fish like salmon, is rich in omega-3 fatty acids, which have heart-protective benefits.

- **Controlling Portion Sizes:** Overeating can lead to weight gain, increasing the risk of heart disease. Practicing portion control and mindful eating can help maintain a healthy weight.

2. Lifestyle and Heart Disease:

- **Regular Physical Activity:** Exercise strengthens the heart muscle, improves circulation, and helps manage weight. The American Heart Association recommends at least 150 minutes of moderate-intensity aerobic activity or 75 minutes of vigorous activity per week, along with muscle-strengthening activities on two or more days per week.

- **Smoking Cessation:** Smoking is a significant risk factor for heart disease. Quitting smoking can dramatically reduce the risk and improve overall heart health. Various resources and support systems are available to help individuals quit smoking.

- **Stress Management:** Chronic stress can negatively impact heart health by increasing blood pressure and leading to unhealthy coping mechanisms such as overeating or smoking. Techniques such as mindfulness, meditation, deep breathing exercises, and regular physical activity can help manage stress.

- **Regular Medical Check-Ups:** Regular check-ups with a healthcare provider can help monitor and manage risk factors for heart disease. This includes blood pressure checks, cholesterol tests, and diabetes screening.

- **Healthy Sleep Patterns:** Poor sleep quality and duration are associated with an increased risk of heart disease. Establishing a regular sleep schedule and creating a restful sleeping environment can improve sleep quality.

Adopting these dietary and lifestyle changes can significantly improve heart health and reduce the risk of complications. The recipes and meal plans in this book are designed to help you make these changes in a practical and enjoyable way.

Explanation of Common Medical Terms Related to Heart Disease

Understanding medical terms related to heart disease can help you better navigate your diagnosis and treatment. Here are some common terms and their explanations:

1. Angina:

- **Definition:** Angina is chest pain or discomfort caused by reduced blood flow to the heart muscle.

- **Types:** Stable angina occurs predictably with exertion and is relieved by rest. Unstable angina is unpredictable, occurs at rest, and may signal an impending heart attack.

2. Atherosclerosis:

- **Definition:** Atherosclerosis is the buildup of fatty deposits (plaque) on the walls of arteries, which can restrict blood flow.

- **Impact:** It can lead to conditions such as CAD, PAD, and stroke.

3. Blood Pressure:

- **Definition:** Blood pressure is the force exerted by blood against the walls of arteries.

- **Components:** It is measured as systolic pressure (the pressure when the heart beats) over diastolic pressure (the pressure when the heart is at rest). Normal blood pressure is around 120/80 mm Hg.

4. Cholesterol:

- **Definition:** Cholesterol is a waxy substance found in blood. While the body needs cholesterol to build healthy cells, high levels can increase the risk of heart disease.

- **Types:** Low-density lipoprotein (LDL) is known as "bad" cholesterol because it can lead to plaque buildup in arteries. High-density lipoprotein (HDL) is known as "good" cholesterol because it helps remove LDL from the bloodstream.

5. Congestive Heart Failure (CHF):

- **Definition:** CHF is a condition in which the heart's ability to pump blood is inadequate to meet the body's needs.

- **Symptoms:** Symptoms include shortness of breath, swelling, and fatigue.

6. Coronary Arteries:

- **Definition:** Coronary arteries are the blood vessels that supply oxygen-rich blood to the heart muscle.

- **Significance:** Blockages or narrowing in these arteries can lead to angina or heart attacks.

7. Electrocardiogram (ECG or EKG):

- **Definition:** An ECG is a test that measures the electrical activity of the heart.

- **Purpose:** It helps diagnose arrhythmias, heart attacks, and other heart conditions.

8. Heart Attack (Myocardial Infarction):

- **Definition:** A heart attack occurs when blood flow to a part of the heart is blocked, causing damage to the heart muscle.

- **Symptoms:** Symptoms include chest pain, shortness of breath, nausea, and lightheadedness.

9. Hypertension:

- **Definition:** Hypertension, or high blood pressure, is a condition where the force of the blood against the artery walls is consistently too high.

- **Risk Factor:** It is a significant risk factor for heart disease, stroke, and kidney disease.

10. Plaque:

- **Definition:** Plaque is a mixture of fatty substances, cholesterol, waste products, and calcium that can build up on the inner walls of arteries.

- **Impact:** Plaque buildup can narrow arteries and reduce blood flow, leading to atherosclerosis.

11. Stent:

- **Definition:** A stent is a small, mesh tube inserted into an artery to keep it open.

- **Purpose:** It is often used to treat narrowed or blocked coronary arteries.

12. Thrombosis:

- **Definition:** Thrombosis is the formation of a blood clot inside a blood vessel, obstructing the flow of blood.

- **Types:** Deep vein thrombosis (DVT) occurs in deep veins, usually in the legs. Coronary thrombosis can cause a heart attack.

13. Triglycerides:

- **Definition:** Triglycerides are a type of fat found in the blood. High levels can increase the risk of heart disease.

- **Management:** Managing triglyceride levels involves diet changes, regular exercise, and sometimes medication.

14. Ventricular Fibrillation:

- **Definition:** Ventricular fibrillation is a life-threatening arrhythmia where the heart's ventricles quiver instead of pumping blood effectively.

- **Emergency:** It requires immediate medical attention, often treated with defibrillation.

By understanding these terms and the role of diet and lifestyle in managing heart disease, you can make informed decisions about your health and work effectively with your healthcare team. This knowledge is the foundation for the recipes and meal plans provided in this book, empowering you to take control of your heart health through delicious, heart-healthy eating.

Chapter 1: The Basics of Heart-Healthy Eating

Key Nutrients for Heart Health

A heart-healthy diet focuses on incorporating a variety of essential nutrients that support cardiovascular health. Understanding these nutrients and the foods that provide them can help you make informed choices about your diet.

1. Fiber:

- **Explanation:** Dietary fiber is crucial for heart health, primarily because it helps lower cholesterol levels and maintain a healthy weight. There are two types of fiber: soluble and insoluble. Soluble fiber dissolves in water and helps reduce blood cholesterol and glucose levels. Insoluble fiber helps move material through your digestive system.

- **Foods Rich in Fiber:**

    o **Fruits:** Apples, oranges, bananas, strawberries, raspberries

    o **Vegetables:** Carrots, beets, broccoli, spinach, Brussels sprouts

    o **Whole Grains:** Oats, barley, brown rice, quinoa, whole wheat bread

- o **Legumes:** Lentils, black beans, chickpeas, kidney beans

- o **Nuts and Seeds:** Almonds, flaxseeds, chia seeds, walnuts

2. Omega-3 Fatty Acids:

- **Explanation:** Omega-3 fatty acids are a type of unsaturated fat that reduce inflammation and lower the risk of chronic diseases such as heart disease. They are particularly effective at lowering triglyceride levels, reducing blood pressure, and preventing blood clots.

- **Foods Rich in Omega-3 Fatty Acids:**

  - o **Fish:** Salmon, mackerel, sardines, trout, herring

  - o **Nuts and Seeds:** Walnuts, flaxseeds, chia seeds, hemp seeds

  - o **Plant Oils:** Flaxseed oil, soybean oil, canola oil

  - o **Other Sources:** Edamame, seaweed, algae supplements

3. Antioxidants:

- **Explanation:** Antioxidants help protect the body from oxidative stress and inflammation, which can damage the arteries and lead to heart disease. Key antioxidants include vitamins C and E, selenium, and flavonoids.

- **Foods Rich in Antioxidants:**

    o **Fruits:** Berries (blueberries, strawberries, blackberries), citrus fruits, apples, grapes

    o **Vegetables:** Kale, spinach, bell peppers, carrots, sweet potatoes

    o **Nuts and Seeds:** Almonds, sunflower seeds, Brazil nuts

    o **Whole Grains:** Oats, barley, quinoa

    o **Beverages:** Green tea, black tea, coffee

4. Potassium:

- **Explanation:** Potassium helps regulate blood pressure by counteracting the effects of sodium. It is crucial for maintaining proper heart function and reducing the risk of stroke.

- **Foods Rich in Potassium:**

    o **Fruits:** Bananas, oranges, apricots, cantaloupe

    o **Vegetables:** Spinach, potatoes, sweet potatoes, tomatoes

    o **Dairy Products:** Milk, yogurt

    o **Fish:** Salmon, tuna, halibut

    o **Other Sources:** Beans, lentils, nuts, seeds

5. Magnesium:

- **Explanation:** Magnesium helps maintain normal muscle and nerve function, keeps the heart rhythm steady, supports a healthy immune system, and keeps bones strong. It also helps regulate blood sugar levels and promotes normal blood pressure.

- **Foods Rich in Magnesium:**
  - **Leafy Greens:** Spinach, Swiss chard, kale
  - **Nuts and Seeds:** Almonds, cashews, pumpkin seeds
  - **Whole Grains:** Brown rice, oats, barley
  - **Legumes:** Black beans, chickpeas, lentils
  - **Fish:** Mackerel, salmon, halibut

6. Healthy Fats:

- **Explanation:** Healthy fats, such as monounsaturated and polyunsaturated fats, can help reduce bad cholesterol levels in your blood, which can lower your risk of heart disease and stroke.

- **Foods Rich in Healthy Fats:**
  - **Oils:** Olive oil, canola oil, sunflower oil
  - **Nuts and Seeds:** Almonds, walnuts, flaxseeds, chia seeds

- Avocados: Rich in monounsaturated fats

- Fatty Fish: Salmon, mackerel, sardines

- Other Sources: Soy products, tofu, edamame

Foods to Avoid

To maintain a heart-healthy diet, it is crucial to limit or avoid certain foods that can negatively impact your heart health. These include foods high in saturated fats, trans fats, sodium, and added sugars.

1. Saturated Fats:

- **Explanation:** Saturated fats can raise your LDL (bad) cholesterol levels, which can increase your risk of heart disease and stroke.

- **Foods High in Saturated Fats:**

  - **Animal Products:** Fatty cuts of meat, poultry with skin, full-fat dairy products (butter, cheese, cream)

  - **Processed Foods:** Baked goods, pastries, doughnuts, cookies

  - **Fast Foods:** Burgers, fried chicken, French fries

2. Trans Fats:

- **Explanation:** Trans fats are particularly harmful because they raise LDL cholesterol levels and lower HDL (good) cholesterol levels. They also increase inflammation and contribute to insulin resistance.

- **Foods High in Trans Fats:**
    - ○ **Processed Foods:** Margarines, shortening, partially hydrogenated oils
    - ○ **Snack Foods:** Chips, crackers, microwave popcorn
    - ○ **Baked Goods:** Cakes, pies, cookies

3. High Sodium:

- **Explanation:** Excessive sodium intake can lead to high blood pressure, a significant risk factor for heart disease and stroke.

- **Foods High in Sodium:**
    - ○ **Processed Foods:** Canned soups, packaged snacks, frozen dinners
    - ○ **Restaurant Meals:** Especially fast food and takeout
    - ○ **Condiments:** Soy sauce, ketchup, salad dressings

4. Added Sugars:

- **Explanation:** High intake of added sugars can lead to obesity, inflammation, high triglyceride levels, and increased risk of heart disease.

- **Foods High in Added Sugars:**

- o **Beverages:** Sodas, energy drinks, sweetened coffee and tea

- o **Sweets:** Candy, cookies, cakes, ice cream

- o **Processed Foods:** Breakfast cereals, granola bars, flavored yogurt

Reading Food Labels and Ingredient Lists

Reading food labels and ingredient lists is essential for making heart-healthy choices. Here are some tips to help you navigate them:

1. Understanding the Nutrition Facts Label:

- **Serving Size:** Check the serving size and compare it to how much you actually eat. Nutritional information is based on this amount.

- **Calories:** Pay attention to the number of calories per serving.

- **Fats:** Look for total fat, saturated fat, and trans fat. Choose products with lower amounts of saturated and trans fats.

- **Cholesterol:** Aim for lower cholesterol levels.

- **Sodium:** Choose foods with lower sodium content.

- **Carbohydrates:** Focus on total carbohydrates, dietary fiber, and sugars. Higher fiber and lower added sugars are preferable.

- **Proteins:** Consider the protein content, especially from plant-based sources.

- **Vitamins and Minerals:** Check for essential nutrients like vitamin D, calcium, iron, and potassium.

2. Ingredients List:

- **Order of Ingredients:** Ingredients are listed in descending order by weight. The first few ingredients are the most prominent.

- **Whole Foods:** Look for whole foods and recognizable ingredients.

- **Added Sugars:** Identify added sugars, which can appear under various names such as high fructose corn syrup, cane sugar, agave nectar, and molasses.

- **Fats and Oils:** Look for healthier oils like olive oil and avoid hydrogenated or partially hydrogenated oils.

- **Sodium:** Check for high-sodium ingredients like salt, sodium benzoate, and monosodium glutamate (MSG).

Building a Balanced Plate

Creating balanced meals is essential for maintaining heart health. This involves portion control, variety, and moderation.

1. Portion Control and Balanced Meals:

- **Understanding Portion Sizes:** Proper portion sizes help control calorie intake and maintain a healthy weight. Use measuring cups, food scales, and portion control plates to manage portions.

- **The Plate Method:** Use the plate method to create balanced meals:

  - **Half Plate with Vegetables and Fruits:** Fill half your plate with a variety of colorful vegetables and fruits.

  - **Quarter Plate with Whole Grains:** Fill one-quarter of your plate with whole grains such as brown rice, quinoa, or whole wheat pasta.

  - **Quarter Plate with Lean Protein:** Fill the remaining quarter with lean protein sources like fish, skinless poultry, beans, or tofu.

- **Healthy Fats:** Include a small amount of healthy fats from sources like avocados, nuts, seeds, or olive oil.

- **Dairy or Dairy Alternatives:** Add a serving of low-fat or fat-free dairy or fortified plant-based alternatives.

2. The Importance of Variety and Moderation:

- **Variety:** Eating a wide range of foods ensures you get all the essential nutrients your body needs. Aim to include different colors, types, and textures of foods in your diet.

- **Moderation:** Even healthy foods can contribute to weight gain if consumed in excess. Practice moderation by listening to your hunger and fullness cues and avoiding overeating.

- **Mindful Eating:** Pay attention to what and how much you eat. Avoid distractions like TV or smartphones during meals, and savor each bite.

3. Practical Tips for Balanced Eating:

- **Meal Planning:** Plan your meals and snacks ahead of time to ensure they are balanced and nutritious.

- **Healthy Snacks:** Choose heart-healthy snacks like fresh fruits, vegetables with hummus, or a handful of nuts.

- **Hydration:** Drink plenty of water throughout the day and limit sugary beverages.

- **Cooking at Home:** Prepare meals at home to have control over ingredients and portion sizes.

Experiment with heart-healthy cooking methods like grilling, steaming, and baking.

By focusing on key nutrients, avoiding harmful foods, and building balanced meals, you can create a heart-healthy eating pattern that supports your overall well-being. The following chapters will provide delicious recipes and practical tips to help you implement these principles in your daily life.

Chapter 2: Meal Planning and Grocery Shopping

Creating a Heart-Healthy Meal Plan

Creating a heart-healthy meal plan is a proactive way to ensure that you consistently consume nutritious meals that support cardiovascular health. This chapter will guide you through crafting a weekly meal plan, offer sample meal plans, and provide tips for effective meal prepping and planning.

1. Sample Weekly Meal Plans:

A balanced meal plan includes a variety of foods that provide essential nutrients. Below are sample meal plans for a week, featuring breakfast, lunch, dinner, and snacks.

Day 1:

- **Breakfast:** Oatmeal topped with fresh berries, a tablespoon of chia seeds, and a drizzle of honey.

- **Lunch:** Quinoa salad with mixed greens, cherry tomatoes, cucumbers, chickpeas, and a lemon-tahini dressing.

- **Dinner:** Grilled salmon with a side of steamed broccoli and a sweet potato.

- **Snacks:** A small apple with almond butter; carrot sticks with hummus.

Day 2:

- **Breakfast:** Smoothie made with spinach, banana, frozen berries, Greek yogurt, and a splash of almond milk.

- **Lunch:** Whole grain wrap with turkey, avocado, spinach, and mustard.

- **Dinner:** Stir-fried tofu with bell peppers, snap peas, and brown rice.

- **Snacks:** Handful of mixed nuts; sliced bell peppers with guacamole.

Day 3:

- **Breakfast:** Whole grain toast with avocado and a poached egg.

- **Lunch:** Lentil soup with a side salad of mixed greens, cucumbers, and vinaigrette.

- **Dinner:** Baked chicken breast with quinoa and roasted Brussels sprouts.

- **Snacks:** A pear; Greek yogurt with a drizzle of honey and a few walnuts.

Day 4:

- **Breakfast:** Greek yogurt parfait with granola, fresh berries, and a sprinkle of flax seeds.

- **Lunch:** Chickpea and vegetable stir-fry with brown rice.

- **Dinner:** Spaghetti squash with marinara sauce and a side of sautéed spinach.

- **Snacks:** An orange; cucumber slices with tzatziki.

Day 5:

- **Breakfast:** Smoothie bowl topped with sliced banana, blueberries, and granola.

- **Lunch:** Mixed bean salad with avocado, cherry tomatoes, corn, and lime dressing.

- **Dinner:** Baked cod with a side of quinoa and roasted asparagus.

- **Snacks:** A handful of trail mix; celery sticks with almond butter.

Day 6:

- **Breakfast:** Whole grain pancakes topped with fresh fruit and a dollop of Greek yogurt.

- **Lunch:** Turkey and avocado salad with mixed greens, cherry tomatoes, and balsamic vinaigrette.

- **Dinner:** Veggie burger on a whole grain bun with a side of sweet potato fries.

- **Snacks:** A kiwi; baby carrots with hummus.

Day 7:

- **Breakfast:** Chia seed pudding made with almond milk, topped with sliced almonds and fresh berries.

- **Lunch:** Quinoa and black bean salad with corn, red bell pepper, and cilantro lime dressing.

- **Dinner:** Grilled shrimp with a side of wild rice and sautéed green beans.

- **Snacks:** A small apple; Greek yogurt with honey and a sprinkle of cinnamon.

2. Tips for Meal Prepping and Planning:

Effective meal prepping and planning can save time, reduce stress, and help you stick to a heart-healthy diet.

A. Plan Ahead:

- **Weekly Planning:** Dedicate time each week to plan your meals. Consider your schedule and choose recipes that fit your lifestyle.

- **Recipe Selection:** Choose a variety of recipes that incorporate different foods to ensure a balanced intake of nutrients.

- **Grocery List:** Create a detailed grocery list based on your meal plan to streamline shopping and avoid impulse purchases.

B. Meal Prepping:

- **Batch Cooking:** Cook larger portions of meals and store them in the refrigerator or freezer for easy access throughout the week.

- **Pre-Cut Vegetables:** Wash and cut vegetables ahead of time to make meal preparation quicker and more convenient.

- **Portion Control:** Use portion control containers to store prepped meals. This helps manage serving sizes and prevents overeating.

- **Labeling:** Label containers with the contents and the date to keep track of freshness and avoid waste.

C. Efficient Cooking:

- **One-Pot Meals:** Opt for one-pot meals like soups, stews, and casseroles that simplify cooking and cleanup.

- **Slow Cooker and Instant Pot:** Utilize slow cookers and Instant Pots for hands-off cooking that can save time and effort.

- **Sheet Pan Dinners:** Prepare sheet pan dinners where you cook all ingredients on a single baking sheet for easy and balanced meals.

D. Healthy Snacking:

- **Nutritious Options:** Keep a stock of healthy snacks like fresh fruit, vegetables with hummus, nuts, and yogurt.

- **Portion Snacks:** Pre-portion snacks into small containers or bags to avoid overeating.

Smart Grocery Shopping

Navigating the grocery store and stocking your pantry, fridge, and freezer with heart-healthy staples are essential steps in maintaining a heart-healthy diet.

1. Navigating the Grocery Store:

A. Shop the Perimeter:

- **Fresh Produce:** Start with the produce section to load up on fresh fruits and vegetables.

- **Lean Proteins:** Move to the meat and seafood sections for lean protein options like chicken, turkey, fish, and plant-based proteins.

- **Dairy and Alternatives:** Choose low-fat or fat-free dairy products or fortified plant-based alternatives.

- **Whole Grains:** Visit the bakery or grains section for whole grain bread, pasta, rice, and oats.

B. Be Cautious in the Aisles:

- **Read Labels:** Carefully read labels on packaged foods to avoid high levels of sodium, added sugars, and unhealthy fats.

- **Frozen Foods:** Choose frozen fruits and vegetables without added sauces or sugars.

These can be just as nutritious as fresh produce and are convenient for meal prepping.

- **Canned Goods:** Select low-sodium or no-salt-added canned vegetables, beans, and fish.

C. Avoid Processed Foods:

- **Minimize Junk Food:** Limit processed snacks, sugary cereals, and high-calorie beverages.

- **Healthier Alternatives:** Opt for healthier snack alternatives like air-popped popcorn, whole grain crackers, and fruit.

2. Heart-Healthy Staples for Your Pantry, Fridge, and Freezer:

A. Pantry Staples:

- **Whole Grains:** Brown rice, quinoa, oats, whole wheat pasta, whole grain bread

- **Legumes:** Canned or dried beans (black beans, chickpeas, lentils), split peas

- **Nuts and Seeds:** Almonds, walnuts, chia seeds, flaxseeds, sunflower seeds

- **Healthy Oils:** Olive oil, canola oil, avocado oil

- **Spices and Herbs:** Dried herbs (basil, oregano, thyme), spices (cumin, turmeric, paprika), garlic powder, onion powder

- **Canned Goods:** Low-sodium or no-salt-added vegetables, tomatoes, and fish (tuna, salmon)

- **Nut Butters:** Natural peanut butter, almond butter

- **Whole Grain Flours:** Whole wheat flour, almond flour, oat flour

B. Fridge Staples:

- **Fresh Produce:** A variety of fruits and vegetables such as berries, apples, oranges, leafy greens, carrots, bell peppers, broccoli

- **Lean Proteins:** Chicken breast, turkey, tofu, tempeh

- **Low-Fat Dairy:** Greek yogurt, low-fat milk, cottage cheese

- **Eggs:** A versatile protein source for breakfast, lunch, or dinner

- **Condiments:** Mustard, salsa, hummus, low-sodium soy sauce, tahini

- **Prepped Items:** Pre-cut vegetables, cooked whole grains, marinated lean proteins for quick meal assembly

C. Freezer Staples:

- **Frozen Vegetables:** Spinach, broccoli, mixed vegetable medleys, peas

- **Frozen Fruits:** Berries, mango, pineapple for smoothies or desserts

- **Lean Proteins:** Fish fillets (salmon, cod), chicken breast, turkey

- **Whole Grains:** Cooked and frozen brown rice, quinoa, whole grain bread

- **Healthy Convenience Items:** Low-sodium vegetable soups, whole grain waffles, veggie burgers

3. Smart Shopping Strategies:

- **Shop with a List:** Always shop with a grocery list based on your meal plan to avoid impulse buying and ensure you get all necessary ingredients.

- **Don't Shop Hungry:** Shopping on an empty stomach can lead to unhealthy impulse purchases. Eat a healthy snack before heading to the store.

- **Compare Labels:** Take the time to compare food labels to choose the healthiest options available.

- **Bulk Buying:** Buy staple items in bulk to save money and ensure you always have essential ingredients on hand.

- **Seasonal Produce:** Choose seasonal fruits and vegetables for better taste, higher nutritional value, and cost savings.

Chapter 3: Breakfast Recipes

Breakfast is an essential meal that sets the tone for the rest of the day. Eating a heart-healthy breakfast can provide you with energy and essential nutrients to start your day off right.

1. Berry Oatmeal

Ingredients:

- 1 cup rolled oats

- 2 cups water or low-fat milk

- 1 cup mixed berries (blueberries, strawberries, raspberries)

- 1 tablespoon chia seeds

- 1 tablespoon honey or maple syrup

- 1 teaspoon cinnamon

Instructions:

1. In a medium saucepan, bring water or milk to a boil.

2. Stir in oats and reduce heat to a simmer.

3. Cook for about 5 minutes, stirring occasionally, until oats are soft.

4. Stir in mixed berries, chia seeds, honey, and cinnamon.

5. Cook for an additional 2 minutes.

6. Serve hot, garnished with extra berries if desired.

Preparation Time: 10 minutes

Nutrition Value (per serving):

- Calories: 250

- Protein: 8g

- Carbohydrates: 45g

- Fiber: 8g

- Total Fat: 5g

- Saturated Fat: 1g

- Sodium: 5mg

2. Avocado and Egg Toast

Ingredients:

- 1 slice whole grain bread

- 1/2 ripe avocado

- 1 egg

- Salt and pepper to taste

- Red pepper flakes (optional)

Instructions:

1. Toast the slice of whole grain bread to your liking.

2. While the bread is toasting, mash the avocado in a small bowl.

3. Spread the mashed avocado evenly over the toast.

4. In a non-stick skillet, cook the egg to your preferred style (fried, scrambled, or poached).

5. Place the cooked egg on top of the avocado toast.

6. Season with salt, pepper, and red pepper flakes if desired.

Preparation Time: 10 minutes

Nutrition Value (per serving):

- Calories: 280

- Protein: 9g

- Carbohydrates: 25g

- Fiber: 7g

- Total Fat: 18g

- Saturated Fat: 3g

- Sodium: 170mg

3. Greek Yogurt Parfait

Ingredients:

- 1 cup Greek yogurt (non-fat or low-fat)

- 1/2 cup granola (low-sugar)

- 1/2 cup fresh berries (blueberries, raspberries, strawberries)

- 1 tablespoon honey

Instructions:

1. In a glass or bowl, layer half of the Greek yogurt.

2. Add half of the granola and fresh berries on top of the yogurt.

3. Repeat the layers with the remaining yogurt, granola, and berries.

4. Drizzle honey over the top before serving.

Preparation Time: 5 minutes

Nutrition Value (per serving):

- Calories: 300

- Protein: 20g

- Carbohydrates: 45g

- Fiber: 6g

- Total Fat: 7g

- Saturated Fat: 2g

- Sodium: 125mg

4. Smoothie Bowl

Ingredients:

- 1 cup spinach

- 1 frozen banana

- 1/2 cup frozen mixed berries

- 1/2 cup unsweetened almond milk

- 1 tablespoon chia seeds

- 1 tablespoon almond butter

- 1/4 cup granola (optional, for topping)

- Fresh fruit slices (optional, for topping)

Instructions:

1. In a blender, combine spinach, frozen banana, mixed berries, almond milk, chia seeds, and almond butter.

2. Blend until smooth and creamy.

3. Pour the smoothie into a bowl.

4. Top with granola and fresh fruit slices if desired.

Preparation Time: 10 minutes

Nutrition Value (per serving):

- Calories: 350

- Protein: 10g

- Carbohydrates: 55g

- Fiber: 12g

- Total Fat: 12g

- Saturated Fat: 1g

- Sodium: 150mg

5. Whole Grain Pancakes

Ingredients:

- 1 cup whole wheat flour

- 1 tablespoon baking powder

- 1 tablespoon honey

- 1 cup low-fat milk or almond milk

- 1 egg

- 1 tablespoon olive oil

- Fresh berries or sliced banana (for topping)

Instructions:

1. In a large bowl, mix whole wheat flour and baking powder.

2. In another bowl, whisk together honey, milk, egg, and olive oil.

3. Pour the wet ingredients into the dry ingredients and stir until just combined.

4. Heat a non-stick skillet over medium heat and lightly grease with oil or cooking spray.

5. Pour 1/4 cup of batter onto the skillet for each pancake.

6. Cook until bubbles form on the surface, then flip and cook until golden brown on both sides.

7. Serve topped with fresh berries or sliced banana.

Preparation Time: 20 minutes

Nutrition Value (per serving, 3 pancakes):

- Calories: 300

- Protein: 10g

- Carbohydrates: 50g

- Fiber: 6g

- Total Fat: 8g

- Saturated Fat: 1g

- Sodium: 380mg

6. Chia Seed Pudding

Ingredients:

- 1/4 cup chia seeds
- 1 cup unsweetened almond milk
- 1 tablespoon honey or maple syrup
- 1/2 teaspoon vanilla extract
- Fresh fruit for topping

Instructions:

1. In a bowl, whisk together chia seeds, almond milk, honey, and vanilla extract.

2. Let the mixture sit for 5 minutes, then whisk again to prevent clumping.

3. Cover and refrigerate for at least 2 hours, or overnight.

4. Stir before serving and top with fresh fruit.

Preparation Time: 5 minutes (plus chilling time)

Nutrition Value (per serving):

- Calories: 200
- Protein: 5g
- Carbohydrates: 25g
- Fiber: 10g
- Total Fat: 10g

- Saturated Fat: 1g

- Sodium: 50mg

7. Spinach and Feta Omelet

Ingredients:

- 3 large eggs or egg whites

- 1 cup fresh spinach

- 1/4 cup crumbled feta cheese

- 1 tablespoon olive oil

- Salt and pepper to taste

Instructions:

1. In a bowl, whisk the eggs and season with salt and pepper.

2. Heat olive oil in a non-stick skillet over medium heat.

3. Add spinach and cook until wilted.

4. Pour the eggs into the skillet and cook until they begin to set.

5. Sprinkle feta cheese over the eggs.

6. Fold the omelet in half and cook until the eggs are fully set.

7. Serve hot.

Preparation Time: 10 minutes

Nutrition Value (per serving):

- Calories: 250
- Protein: 18g
- Carbohydrates: 4g
- Fiber: 1g
- Total Fat: 18g
- Saturated Fat: 6g
- Sodium: 400mg

8. Quinoa Breakfast Bowl

Ingredients:

- 1 cup cooked quinoa
- 1/2 cup almond milk
- 1 tablespoon honey or maple syrup
- 1/2 teaspoon cinnamon
- 1/4 cup fresh berries
- 1 tablespoon chopped nuts (almonds, walnuts)

Instructions:

1. In a small saucepan, warm the cooked quinoa with almond milk over medium heat.
2. Stir in honey and cinnamon.
3. Cook until the mixture is heated through.

4. Serve topped with fresh berries and chopped nuts.

Preparation Time: 10 minutes (using pre-cooked quinoa)

Nutrition Value (per serving):

- Calories: 300

- Protein: 9g

- Carbohydrates: 45g

- Fiber: 6g

- Total Fat: 10g

- Saturated Fat: 1g

- Sodium: 50mg

9. Peanut Butter Banana Smoothie

Ingredients:

- 1 banana

- 1 cup unsweetened almond milk

- 2 tablespoons natural peanut butter

- 1 tablespoon chia seeds

- 1/2 teaspoon vanilla extract

Instructions:

1. Combine all ingredients in a blender.

2. Blend until smooth and creamy.

3. Pour into a glass and enjoy.

Preparation Time: 5 minutes

Nutrition Value (per serving):

- Calories: 300

- Protein: 8g

- Carbohydrates: 40g

- Fiber: 8g

- Total Fat: 15g

- Saturated Fat: 2g

- Sodium: 200mg

10. Sweet Potato and Black Bean Breakfast Burrito

Ingredients:

- 1 small sweet potato, peeled and diced

- 1/2 cup black beans, rinsed and drained

- 1 small avocado, sliced

- 1 tablespoon olive oil

- 1 whole grain tortilla

- Salt and pepper to taste

- Salsa (optional)

Instructions:

1. Heat olive oil in a skillet over medium heat.

2. Add diced sweet potato and cook until tender and lightly browned, about 10 minutes.

3. Add black beans and cook until heated through.

4. Season with salt and pepper.

5. Warm the tortilla in a separate skillet or microwave.

6. Fill the tortilla with the sweet potato and black bean mixture.

7. Add avocado slices and salsa if desired.

8. Roll up the tortilla and serve.

Preparation Time: 20 minutes

Nutrition Value (per serving):

- Calories: 350

- Protein: 9g

- Carbohydrates: 50g

- Fiber: 12g

- Total Fat: 12g

- Saturated Fat: 2g

- Sodium: 300mg

These ten breakfast recipes are designed to provide a variety of delicious, heart-healthy options to start your day with essential nutrients, balanced energy, and great taste

Chapter 4: Lunch Recipes

Lunch is an important meal that helps sustain energy levels and keeps you focused throughout the day.

1. Quinoa and Black Bean Salad

Ingredients:

- 1 cup quinoa, cooked
- 1 cup black beans, rinsed and drained
- 1 cup cherry tomatoes, halved
- 1/2 cup corn kernels
- 1/4 cup red onion, diced
- 1/4 cup cilantro, chopped
- 2 tablespoons olive oil
- 1 tablespoon lime juice
- Salt and pepper to taste

Instructions:

1. In a large bowl, combine cooked quinoa, black beans, cherry tomatoes, corn, red onion, and cilantro.

2. In a small bowl, whisk together olive oil, lime juice, salt, and pepper.

3. Pour the dressing over the salad and toss to combine.

4. Serve immediately or refrigerate for later.

Preparation Time: 15 minutes

Nutrition Value (per serving):

- Calories: 300

- Protein: 10g

- Carbohydrates: 45g

- Fiber: 10g

- Total Fat: 10g

- Saturated Fat: 1g

- Sodium: 250mg

2. Grilled Chicken and Avocado Wrap

Ingredients:

- 1 whole grain tortilla

- 1 grilled chicken breast, sliced

- 1/2 avocado, sliced

- 1/2 cup mixed greens

- 1/4 cup shredded carrots

- 1 tablespoon hummus

Instructions:

1. Spread hummus evenly over the tortilla.

2. Layer with mixed greens, shredded carrots, grilled chicken slices, and avocado slices.

3. Roll up the tortilla tightly and cut in half.

4. Serve immediately.

Preparation Time: 10 minutes

Nutrition Value (per serving):

- Calories: 350

- Protein: 25g

- Carbohydrates: 30g

- Fiber: 10g

- Total Fat: 15g

- Saturated Fat: 2g

- Sodium: 300mg

3. Lentil Soup

Ingredients:

- 1 cup dried lentils, rinsed

- 1 medium onion, diced

- 2 carrots, diced

- 2 celery stalks, diced

- 2 cloves garlic, minced

- 1 can (14.5 oz) diced tomatoes

- 4 cups low-sodium vegetable broth

- 1 teaspoon cumin

- 1 teaspoon thyme

- 1 bay leaf

- 1 tablespoon olive oil

- Salt and pepper to taste

Instructions:

1. In a large pot, heat olive oil over medium heat.

2. Add onion, carrots, celery, and garlic. Sauté until vegetables are tender, about 5 minutes.

3. Add lentils, diced tomatoes, vegetable broth, cumin, thyme, and bay leaf.

4. Bring to a boil, then reduce heat and simmer for 30-35 minutes, or until lentils are tender.

5. Season with salt and pepper to taste.

6. Remove bay leaf before serving.

Preparation Time: 45 minutes

Nutrition Value (per serving):

- Calories: 250

- Protein: 15g

- Carbohydrates: 40g

- Fiber: 15g

- Total Fat: 5g

- Saturated Fat: 1g

- Sodium: 300mg

4. Chickpea and Vegetable Stir-Fry

Ingredients:

- 1 can (15 oz) chickpeas, rinsed and drained

- 1 red bell pepper, sliced

- 1 yellow bell pepper, sliced

- 1 zucchini, sliced

- 1 cup broccoli florets

- 2 cloves garlic, minced

- 2 tablespoons olive oil

- 2 tablespoons low-sodium soy sauce

- 1 tablespoon honey or maple syrup

- 1 teaspoon ginger, minced

- 1 cup cooked brown rice

Instructions:

1. In a large skillet, heat olive oil over medium-high heat.

2. Add garlic and ginger, sauté for 1 minute.

3. Add bell peppers, zucchini, and broccoli. Stir-fry for 5-7 minutes, until vegetables are tender.

4. Add chickpeas, soy sauce, and honey. Stir well and cook for an additional 2-3 minutes.

5. Serve over cooked brown rice.

Preparation Time: 20 minutes

Nutrition Value (per serving):

- Calories: 350

- Protein: 10g

- Carbohydrates: 55g

- Fiber: 12g

- Total Fat: 10g

- Saturated Fat: 1g

- Sodium: 400mg

5. Turkey and Avocado Salad

Ingredients:

- 2 cups mixed greens

- 4 oz cooked turkey breast, sliced

- 1/2 avocado, diced

- 1/4 cup cherry tomatoes, halved

- 1/4 cup cucumber, sliced

- 2 tablespoons olive oil

- 1 tablespoon balsamic vinegar

- Salt and pepper to taste

Instructions:

1. In a large bowl, combine mixed greens, turkey slices, avocado, cherry tomatoes, and cucumber.

2. In a small bowl, whisk together olive oil, balsamic vinegar, salt, and pepper.

3. Pour dressing over the salad and toss to combine.

4. Serve immediately.

Preparation Time: 10 minutes

Nutrition Value (per serving):

- Calories: 300

- Protein: 25g

- Carbohydrates: 15g

- Fiber: 7g

- Total Fat: 18g

- Saturated Fat: 3g

- Sodium: 250mg

6. Mediterranean Pasta Salad

Ingredients:

- 2 cups cooked whole wheat pasta
- 1 cup cherry tomatoes, halved
- 1/2 cup cucumber, diced
- 1/4 cup Kalamata olives, sliced
- 1/4 cup red onion, diced
- 1/4 cup feta cheese, crumbled
- 2 tablespoons olive oil
- 1 tablespoon red wine vinegar
- 1 teaspoon dried oregano
- Salt and pepper to taste

Instructions:

1. In a large bowl, combine cooked pasta, cherry tomatoes, cucumber, olives, red onion, and feta cheese.

2. In a small bowl, whisk together olive oil, red wine vinegar, oregano, salt, and pepper.

3. Pour dressing over the pasta salad and toss to combine.

4. Serve immediately or refrigerate for later.

Preparation Time: 15 minutes

Nutrition Value (per serving):

- Calories: 350
- Protein: 10g
- Carbohydrates: 45g
- Fiber: 7g
- Total Fat: 15g
- Saturated Fat: 4g
- Sodium: 400mg

7. Sweet Potato and Black Bean Tacos

Ingredients:

- 1 medium sweet potato, peeled and diced
- 1 can (15 oz) black beans, rinsed and drained
- 1/2 cup corn kernels
- 1/4 cup red onion, diced
- 1/4 cup cilantro, chopped
- 1 tablespoon olive oil
- 1 teaspoon cumin
- 1 teaspoon chili powder
- Salt and pepper to taste
- 4 whole grain tortillas
- Salsa and avocado slices for serving

Instructions:

1. Preheat oven to 400°F (200°C).

2. Toss sweet potato with olive oil, cumin, chili powder, salt, and pepper. Spread on a baking sheet.

3. Roast for 20-25 minutes, until tender and lightly browned.

4. In a large bowl, combine roasted sweet potato, black beans, corn, red onion, and cilantro.

5. Warm tortillas in a skillet or microwave.

6. Fill each tortilla with the sweet potato and black bean mixture.

7. Serve with salsa and avocado slices.

Preparation Time: 30 minutes

Nutrition Value (per serving):

- Calories: 350

- Protein: 10g

- Carbohydrates: 60g

- Fiber: 12g

- Total Fat: 8g

- Saturated Fat: 1g

- Sodium: 400mg

8. Spinach and Feta Stuffed Peppers

Ingredients:

- 4 bell peppers, halved and seeds removed
- 2 cups cooked brown rice
- 1 cup fresh spinach, chopped
- 1/2 cup feta cheese, crumbled
- 1/4 cup red onion, diced
- 1 clove garlic, minced
- 1 tablespoon olive oil
- Salt and pepper to taste

Instructions:

1. Preheat oven to 375°F (190°C).
2. In a large skillet, heat olive oil over medium heat.
3. Add garlic and red onion, sauté for 2-3 minutes.
4. Add spinach and cook until wilted.
5. In a large bowl, combine cooked rice, spinach mixture, and feta cheese. Season with salt and pepper.
6. Stuff each bell pepper half with the rice mixture.
7. Place stuffed peppers in a baking dish and cover with foil.

8. Bake for 25-30 minutes, until peppers are tender.

Preparation Time: 40 minutes

Nutrition Value (per serving):

- Calories: 300

- Protein: 10g

- Carbohydrates: 45g

- Fiber: 7g

- Total Fat: 10g

- Saturated Fat: 3g

- Sodium: 350mg

9. Tuna Salad Lettuce Wraps

Ingredients:

- 1 can (5 oz) tuna, drained

- 1/4 cup plain Greek yogurt

- 1 tablespoon Dijon mustard

- 1 celery stalk, diced

- 1/4 cup red bell pepper, diced

- 1/4 cup red onion, diced

- 1 tablespoon fresh dill, chopped

- Salt and pepper to taste

- Large lettuce leaves for wrapping

Instructions:

1. In a medium bowl, combine tuna, Greek yogurt, Dijon mustard, celery, bell pepper, red onion, and dill.

2. Season with salt and pepper to taste.

3. Spoon the tuna salad onto large lettuce leaves and wrap.

4. Serve immediately.

Preparation Time: 10 minutes

Nutrition Value (per serving):

- Calories: 200

- Protein: 25g

- Carbohydrates: 10g

- Fiber: 2g

- Total Fat: 7g

- Saturated Fat: 1g

- Sodium: 300mg

10. Veggie and Hummus Sandwich

Ingredients:

- 2 slices whole grain bread

- 1/4 cup hummus

- 1/2 cucumber, sliced
- 1/4 cup shredded carrots
- 1/4 cup bell pepper, sliced
- 1/4 cup spinach leaves
- Salt and pepper to taste

Instructions:

1. Spread hummus evenly over one slice of bread.

2. Layer with cucumber slices, shredded carrots, bell pepper slices, and spinach leaves.

3. Season with salt and pepper.

4. Top with the second slice of bread.

5. Cut in half and serve.

Preparation Time: 10 minutes

Nutrition Value (per serving):

- Calories: 300
- Protein: 10g
- Carbohydrates: 45g
- Fiber: 10g
- Total Fat: 10g
- Saturated Fat: 1g
- Sodium: 350mg

Chapter 5: Dinner Recipes

Dinner is an opportunity to relax and enjoy a nourishing meal that supports heart health.

1. Baked Salmon with Asparagus

Ingredients:

- 4 salmon fillets (about 4 oz each)
- 1 bunch asparagus, trimmed
- 2 tablespoons olive oil
- 2 cloves garlic, minced
- 1 lemon, sliced
- Salt and pepper to taste

Instructions:

1. Preheat oven to 400°F (200°C).
2. Place salmon fillets and asparagus on a baking sheet.
3. Drizzle with olive oil and sprinkle with minced garlic, salt, and pepper.
4. Top with lemon slices.
5. Bake for 15-20 minutes, until salmon is cooked through and asparagus is tender.

Preparation Time: 25 minutes

Nutrition Value (per serving):

- Calories: 350
- Protein: 30g
- Carbohydrates: 5g
- Fiber: 2g
- Total Fat: 22g
- Saturated Fat: 3g
- Sodium: 180mg

2. Quinoa-Stuffed Bell Peppers

Ingredients:

- 4 bell peppers, tops cut off and seeds removed
- 1 cup cooked quinoa
- 1 can (15 oz) black beans, rinsed and drained
- 1 cup corn kernels
- 1 cup diced tomatoes
- 1/2 cup shredded low-fat cheese
- 1 teaspoon cumin
- 1 teaspoon chili powder
- Salt and pepper to taste

Instructions:

1. Preheat oven to 375°F (190°C).

2. In a large bowl, combine cooked quinoa, black beans, corn, diced tomatoes, cumin, chili powder, salt, and pepper.

3. Stuff the bell peppers with the quinoa mixture and place them in a baking dish.

4. Cover with foil and bake for 25 minutes.

5. Remove foil, sprinkle with cheese, and bake for an additional 10 minutes.

Preparation Time: 40 minutes

Nutrition Value (per serving):

- Calories: 300

- Protein: 12g

- Carbohydrates: 50g

- Fiber: 10g

- Total Fat: 8g

- Saturated Fat: 3g

- Sodium: 300mg

3. Lemon Herb Chicken with Roasted Vegetables

Ingredients:

- 4 boneless, skinless chicken breasts

- 1/4 cup olive oil

- 2 lemons, juiced

- 3 cloves garlic, minced

- 1 teaspoon dried oregano

- 1 teaspoon dried thyme

- Salt and pepper to taste

- 1 pound baby potatoes, halved

- 1 cup baby carrots

- 1 red onion, cut into wedges

Instructions:

1. Preheat oven to 400°F (200°C).

2. In a small bowl, whisk together olive oil, lemon juice, garlic, oregano, thyme, salt, and pepper.

3. Place chicken breasts in a baking dish and pour half of the marinade over them.

4. Arrange baby potatoes, carrots, and red onion around the chicken.

5. Drizzle remaining marinade over the vegetables.

6. Bake for 30-35 minutes, until chicken is cooked through and vegetables are tender.

Preparation Time: 45 minutes

Nutrition Value (per serving):

- Calories: 400

- Protein: 35g

- Carbohydrates: 35g

- Fiber: 6g

- Total Fat: 15g

- Saturated Fat: 2g

- Sodium: 200mg

4. Spaghetti Squash with Marinara Sauce

Ingredients:

- 1 medium spaghetti squash

- 2 tablespoons olive oil

- 1 small onion, diced

- 2 cloves garlic, minced

- 1 can (28 oz) crushed tomatoes

- 1 teaspoon dried basil

- 1 teaspoon dried oregano

- 1/4 cup fresh basil, chopped

- Salt and pepper to taste

Instructions:

1. Preheat oven to 375°F (190°C).

2. Cut spaghetti squash in half lengthwise and remove seeds.

3. Place squash halves cut-side down on a baking sheet and bake for 40 minutes.

4. While squash is baking, heat olive oil in a saucepan over medium heat.

5. Add onion and garlic, sauté until soft.

6. Stir in crushed tomatoes, dried basil, dried oregano, salt, and pepper. Simmer for 15-20 minutes.

7. When squash is done, use a fork to scrape out the spaghetti-like strands.

8. Serve the spaghetti squash topped with marinara sauce and fresh basil.

Preparation Time: 50 minutes

Nutrition Value (per serving):

- Calories: 250

- Protein: 5g

- Carbohydrates: 35g

- Fiber: 8g

- Total Fat: 10g

- Saturated Fat: 1g

- Sodium: 400mg

5. Grilled Shrimp Skewers with Veggies

Ingredients:

- 1 pound large shrimp, peeled and deveined
- 1 red bell pepper, cut into chunks
- 1 yellow bell pepper, cut into chunks
- 1 zucchini, sliced
- 1 red onion, cut into chunks
- 2 tablespoons olive oil
- 2 tablespoons lemon juice
- 2 cloves garlic, minced
- Salt and pepper to taste
- Wooden or metal skewers

Instructions:

1. Preheat grill to medium-high heat.
2. In a bowl, combine olive oil, lemon juice, garlic, salt, and pepper.
3. Thread shrimp and vegetables onto skewers.
4. Brush skewers with the olive oil mixture.
5. Grill skewers for 2-3 minutes per side, until shrimp are opaque and vegetables are tender.

Preparation Time: 20 minutes

Nutrition Value (per serving):

- Calories: 250

- Protein: 25g

- Carbohydrates: 10g

- Fiber: 3g

- Total Fat: 12g

- Saturated Fat: 2g

- Sodium: 450mg

6. Turkey Meatballs with Zoodles

Ingredients:

- 1 pound ground turkey

- 1/4 cup whole wheat breadcrumbs

- 1/4 cup grated Parmesan cheese

- 1 egg

- 2 cloves garlic, minced

- 1 teaspoon dried oregano

- 1 teaspoon dried basil

- Salt and pepper to taste

- 2 tablespoons olive oil

- 4 zucchini, spiralized into noodles

- 1 cup marinara sauce

Instructions:

1. In a large bowl, combine ground turkey, breadcrumbs, Parmesan cheese, egg, garlic, oregano, basil, salt, and pepper.

2. Form mixture into meatballs.

3. Heat olive oil in a skillet over medium heat.

4. Cook meatballs until browned and cooked through, about 10 minutes.

5. In another skillet, sauté zucchini noodles for 2-3 minutes, until just tender.

6. Serve meatballs over zucchini noodles with marinara sauce.

Preparation Time: 30 minutes

Nutrition Value (per serving):

- Calories: 350

- Protein: 30g

- Carbohydrates: 20g

- Fiber: 6g

- Total Fat: 18g

- Saturated Fat: 4g

- Sodium: 450mg

7. Baked Cod with Tomatoes and Olives

Ingredients:

- 4 cod fillets (about 4 oz each)
- 2 cups cherry tomatoes, halved
- 1/2 cup Kalamata olives, sliced
- 1/4 cup red onion, diced
- 2 tablespoons olive oil
- 2 cloves garlic, minced
- 1 teaspoon dried oregano
- Salt and pepper to taste

Instructions:

1. Preheat oven to 400°F (200°C).
2. In a baking dish, combine cherry tomatoes, olives, red onion, olive oil, garlic, oregano, salt, and pepper.
3. Place cod fillets on top of the tomato mixture.
4. Bake for 20-25 minutes, until cod is cooked through and flakes easily with a fork.

Preparation Time: 30 minutes

Nutrition Value (per serving):

- Calories: 300
- Protein: 30g
- Carbohydrates: 10g

- Fiber: 3g

- Total Fat: 15g

- Saturated Fat: 2g

- Sodium: 400mg

8. Vegetable Stir-Fry with Tofu

Ingredients:

- 1 block (14 oz) firm tofu, drained and cubed

- 1 red bell pepper, sliced

- 1 yellow bell pepper, sliced

- 1 cup broccoli florets

- 1 carrot, julienned

- 2 tablespoons soy sauce (low-sodium)

- 1 tablespoon sesame oil

- 2 cloves garlic, minced

- 1 teaspoon ginger, minced

- 2 tablespoons olive oil

Instructions:

1. Heat olive oil in a large skillet over medium-high heat.

2. Add tofu cubes and cook until golden brown, about 5-7 minutes. Remove and set aside.

3. In the same skillet, add sesame oil, garlic, and ginger. Sauté for 1 minute.

4. Add bell peppers, broccoli, and carrot. Stir-fry for 5-7 minutes, until vegetables are tender.

5. Return tofu to the skillet and add soy sauce. Stir well to combine.

6. Serve immediately.

Preparation Time: 20 minutes

Nutrition Value (per serving):

- Calories: 300

- Protein: 15g

- Carbohydrates: 20g

- Fiber: 6g

- Total Fat: 18g

- Saturated Fat: 2g

- Sodium: 350mg

9. Lentil and Vegetable Curry

Ingredients:

- 1 cup dried lentils, rinsed

- 1 onion, diced

- 2 cloves garlic, minced

- 1 tablespoon ginger, minced

- 1 can (14.5 oz) diced tomatoes
- 1 can (14 oz) coconut milk (light)
- 1 cup vegetable broth
- 1 cup spinach, chopped
- 1 tablespoon curry powder
- 1 teaspoon cumin
- 2 tablespoons olive oil
- Salt and pepper to taste

Instructions:

1. In a large pot, heat olive oil over medium heat.
2. Add onion, garlic, and ginger. Sauté until fragrant, about 5 minutes.
3. Stir in curry powder and cumin, cooking for another minute.
4. Add lentils, diced tomatoes, coconut milk, and vegetable broth. Bring to a boil.
5. Reduce heat and simmer for 25-30 minutes, until lentils are tender.
6. Stir in spinach and cook until wilted.
7. Season with salt and pepper to taste.

Preparation Time: 35 minutes

Nutrition Value (per serving):

- Calories: 350

- Protein: 15g

- Carbohydrates: 45g

- Fiber: 15g

- Total Fat: 12g

- Saturated Fat: 4g

- Sodium: 400mg

10. Baked Chicken with Brussels Sprouts and Sweet Potatoes

Ingredients:

- 4 boneless, skinless chicken breasts

- 1 pound Brussels sprouts, halved

- 2 medium sweet potatoes, diced

- 2 tablespoons olive oil

- 2 cloves garlic, minced

- 1 teaspoon dried thyme

- Salt and pepper to taste

Instructions:

1. Preheat oven to 400°F (200°C).

2. Place chicken breasts, Brussels sprouts, and sweet potatoes on a baking sheet.

3. Drizzle with olive oil and sprinkle with minced garlic, thyme, salt, and pepper.

4. Toss to coat evenly.

5. Bake for 25-30 minutes, until chicken is cooked through and vegetables are tender.

Preparation Time: 35 minutes

Nutrition Value (per serving):

- Calories: 400

- Protein: 35g

- Carbohydrates: 35g

- Fiber: 7g

- Total Fat: 15g

- Saturated Fat: 2g

- Sodium: 200mg

CHAPTER 6: SNACKS RECIPES

1. Avocado Toast

Ingredients:

- 1 ripe avocado
- 2 slices whole-grain bread
- 1 tablespoon lemon juice
- Salt and pepper to taste
- Optional: cherry tomatoes, red pepper flakes

Instructions:

1. Toast the whole-grain bread.
2. Mash the avocado in a bowl and add lemon juice, salt, and pepper.
3. Spread the avocado mixture on the toasted bread.
4. Top with cherry tomatoes and red pepper flakes if desired.

Preparation Time: 10 minutes

Nutrition Value (per serving):

- Calories: 220
- Fat: 14g

- Carbohydrates: 22g

- Protein: 4g

- Fiber: 8g

2. Greek Yogurt with Berries

Ingredients:

- 1 cup Greek yogurt (non-fat)

- 1/2 cup mixed berries (blueberries, strawberries, raspberries)

- 1 tablespoon honey

- 1 tablespoon chia seeds

Instructions:

1. In a bowl, combine Greek yogurt and honey.

2. Top with mixed berries and chia seeds.

Preparation Time: 5 minutes

Nutrition Value (per serving):

- Calories: 150

- Fat: 2g

- Carbohydrates: 20g

- Protein: 14g

- Fiber: 5g

3. Hummus and Veggie Sticks

Ingredients:

- 1 cup hummus
- 1 carrot, cut into sticks
- 1 cucumber, cut into sticks
- 1 bell pepper, cut into sticks

Instructions:

1. Arrange the vegetable sticks on a plate.
2. Serve with a bowl of hummus.

Preparation Time: 10 minutes

Nutrition Value (per serving):

- Calories: 180
- Fat: 8g
- Carbohydrates: 22g
- Protein: 6g
- Fiber: 8g

4. Apple Slices with Almond Butter

Ingredients:

- 1 apple, sliced
- 2 tablespoons almond butter

Instructions:

1. Core and slice the apple.

2. Serve with almond butter for dipping.

Preparation Time: 5 minutes

Nutrition Value (per serving):

- Calories: 210

- Fat: 14g

- Carbohydrates: 22g

- Protein: 4g

- Fiber: 6g

5. Edamame

Ingredients:

- 1 cup edamame (in pods or shelled)

- Salt to taste

Instructions:

1. Boil or steam the edamame according to package instructions.

2. Sprinkle with salt to taste.

Preparation Time: 10 minutes

Nutrition Value (per serving):

- Calories: 120

- Fat: 5g

- Carbohydrates: 9g

- Protein: 11g

- Fiber: 4g

6. Oatmeal Energy Balls

Ingredients:

- 1 cup rolled oats

- 1/2 cup peanut butter

- 1/3 cup honey

- 1/4 cup dark chocolate chips

- 1/4 cup flaxseeds

Instructions:

1. Combine all ingredients in a bowl and mix well.

2. Roll into small balls and refrigerate for 30 minutes before serving.

Preparation Time: 10 minutes + 30 minutes refrigeration

Nutrition Value (per serving, 2 balls):

- Calories: 200

- Fat: 10g

- Carbohydrates: 25g

- Protein: 5g

- Fiber: 4g

7. Mixed Nuts

Ingredients:

- 1/4 cup mixed unsalted nuts (almonds, walnuts, cashews)

Instructions:

1. Serve mixed nuts in a small bowl.

Preparation Time: 1 minute

Nutrition Value (per serving):

- Calories: 200

- Fat: 18g

- Carbohydrates: 6g

- Protein: 6g

- Fiber: 4g

8. Cottage Cheese with Pineapple

Ingredients:

- 1 cup low-fat cottage cheese

- 1/2 cup pineapple chunks (fresh or canned in juice, drained)

Instructions:

1. Combine cottage cheese and pineapple chunks in a bowl.

Preparation Time: 5 minutes

Nutrition Value (per serving):

- Calories: 150

- Fat: 2g

- Carbohydrates: 16g

- Protein: 16g

- Fiber: 2g

9. Kale Chips

Ingredients:

- 1 bunch kale, washed and torn into pieces

- 1 tablespoon olive oil

- Salt to taste

Instructions:

1. Preheat oven to 350°F (175°C).

2. Toss the kale with olive oil and salt.

3. Spread on a baking sheet and bake for 10-15 minutes until crispy.

Preparation Time: 20 minutes

Nutrition Value (per serving):

- Calories: 80

- Fat: 4g

- Carbohydrates: 10g

- Protein: 3g
- Fiber: 3g

10. Chia Pudding

Ingredients:

- 1 cup almond milk
- 3 tablespoons chia seeds
- 1 tablespoon maple syrup
- 1/2 teaspoon vanilla extract

Instructions:

1. Combine all ingredients in a bowl and mix well.
2. Refrigerate for at least 2 hours or overnight.

Preparation Time: 5 minutes + 2 hours refrigeration

Nutrition Value (per serving):

- Calories: 150
- Fat: 8g
- Carbohydrates: 16g
- Protein: 4g
- Fiber: 10g

CONCLUSION

It's important to reflect on the journey we've embarked on together. Throughout these pages, we've explored the intricate relationship between diet and heart health, delved into the science behind nutrition, and uncovered the power of whole, plant-based foods to heal and rejuvenate our cardiovascular system. This book is more than a collection of recipes; it's a roadmap to a healthier, more vibrant life.

The Power of Food as Medicine

The recipes and meal plans we've shared are built upon the foundational principle that food is medicine. Each ingredient, each dish, is carefully selected and crafted to provide the maximum benefit to your heart. The antioxidants in berries, the healthy fats in avocados, the fiber in whole grains—all these components work synergistically to reduce inflammation, lower cholesterol levels, and improve blood flow.

The scientific community has increasingly recognized the profound impact of diet on heart disease. Studies have consistently shown that plant-based diets can not only prevent but also reverse the progression of heart disease. By eliminating or significantly reducing animal products and processed foods, and instead focusing on fruits, vegetables, legumes, nuts, and seeds, we provide our bodies with the nutrients they need to thrive.

Empowering Yourself with Knowledge

Knowledge is a powerful tool in the fight against heart disease. By understanding how different foods affect our cardiovascular health, we can make informed choices that support our well-being. This book has aimed to demystify the complexities of nutrition and provide clear, actionable advice.

We've discussed the role of cholesterol and saturated fats, the dangers of added sugars and refined carbohydrates, and the benefits of dietary fiber and antioxidants. Armed with this information, you are now better equipped to navigate the often confusing world of nutrition and make choices that align with your health goals.

Practical Tips for Lasting Change

Adopting a heart-healthy diet is a journey, not a destination. It's about making sustainable changes that become a natural part of your lifestyle. Here are some practical tips to help you continue on this path:

1. **Start Small:** Begin by incorporating one or two new recipes into your weekly meal plan. Gradually increase the number as you become more comfortable with the ingredients and cooking techniques.

2. **Plan Ahead:** Take some time each week to plan your meals and snacks. Having a plan reduces the temptation to reach for unhealthy options.

3. **Keep It Simple:** Healthy eating doesn't have to be complicated. Focus on simple, whole foods and let the natural flavors shine through.

4. **Listen to Your Body:** Pay attention to how different foods make you feel. Everyone's body is unique, and it's important to find what works best for you.

5. **Stay Hydrated:** Water is essential for overall health, including heart health. Aim to drink plenty of water throughout the day.

The Role of Community and Support

Embarking on a journey to reverse heart disease can feel daunting, but you don't have to do it alone. Seek support from friends, family, or a community of like-minded individuals who share your goals. Share your successes and challenges, exchange recipes, and encourage each other along the way.

Joining a cooking class or a nutrition group can also be a great way to stay motivated and learn new skills. Remember, every step you take towards a healthier diet is a victory worth celebrating.

Beyond the Kitchen: Holistic Heart Health

While diet plays a crucial role in heart health, it's just one piece of the puzzle. A holistic approach to heart health also includes regular physical activity, stress management, and adequate sleep.

1. **Exercise:** Aim for at least 150 minutes of moderate-intensity exercise each week. Find activities you enjoy, whether it's walking, cycling, swimming, or dancing.

2. **Stress Management:** Chronic stress can negatively impact heart health. Incorporate stress-reducing practices into your daily routine, such as meditation, yoga, or deep breathing exercises.

3. **Sleep:** Quality sleep is essential for overall health. Aim for 7-9 hours of sleep per night and establish a consistent sleep schedule.

Celebrating Progress and Looking Forward

As you continue on your journey to better heart health, take time to celebrate your progress. Every positive change, no matter how small, is a step in the right direction. Reflect on how far you've come and the improvements you've noticed in your health and well-being.

Looking forward, remember that the journey to heart health is ongoing. Stay curious, keep experimenting with new recipes, and continue to educate yourself about nutrition and health. The knowledge and habits you've gained through this book will serve you well for years to come.

A Call to Action

Now, it's time to take action. You've armed yourself with the knowledge, the recipes, and the motivation.

The next step is to put it all into practice. Start today—make a heart-healthy meal, go for a walk, meditate for a few minutes. Every action counts.

Share your journey with others. Inspire your friends and family to join you in embracing a heart-healthy lifestyle. By making positive changes in your own life, you can create a ripple effect that extends far beyond yourself.

Gratitude and Final Thoughts

In closing, we want to express our gratitude for joining us on this journey. Your commitment to improving your heart health is commendable, and we are honored to be a part of it. We hope that the book has provided you with the tools, knowledge, and inspiration to transform your diet and your life.